BORDERLINE PERSONALITY DISORDER DEMYSTIFIED

A COMPLETE SURVIVAL GUIDE TO LOVING SOMEONE WITH BORDERLINE PERSONALITY DISORDER

LINSY B.

© 2019 Linsy B.

You are welcome to join the Fan's Corner, here

Disclaimer

Dedication

This work is dedicated to Oje and Sem, without whose help, this book would not have come to light.

Table of Content

Introduction

Loneliness is a situation we all suffer from at different stages of our lives, but no one fears the feeling of being alone as much as a person with a borderline personality disorder. A mental health disorder that makes the victim have intense moments of love in which they see their loved one as a perfect individual only to change their opinion suddenly about the same person.

Fluctuating between this pattern of idealizing their loved ones to then devaluating them, a BPD displays an incoherent behavior that makes it difficult for anyone to be their friend for too long. They react to the possibility of being abandoned by threatening and actually harming themselves, indulging in risky sexual activities, drug abuse, and excessive shopping. If you are involved with them, you will also have had to deal with situations where they contemplate and attempt suicide.

Loving someone who has a borderline personality disorder is not an easy thing to do. They will leave you emotionally drained, insecure and paranoia, which is why you have to take steps to protect yourself so that you do not also relapse into becoming a mental health patient.

Understanding Borderline Personality Disorder

People with Borderline personality disorder (BPD) usually react strongly to a real or perceived belief they are about to be abandoned by their loved ones which could make them become lonely. The key to understanding borderline personality disorder people is to research by reading borderline personality disorder books that talk about the different aspects of BPD. If you have BPD kids, parents, friends or lovers, you will become aware of the trauma living with them, which is why a sort of borderline personality disorder survival guide or an essential family guide such as this one can become very useful.

The fear of suffering from loneliness as a result of being abandoned by loved ones is a major prevailing fear in the mind of every BPD, which can reach such intensity that can warrant them hurting themselves in order to get back the attention and affection of their loved one. Psychologists are always concerned about the effects of loneliness and depression, which can lead to a lot of other mental and physical health issues.

The Concept of Loneliness

To be lonely is to feel alone, isolated and away from others. It is a physical and psychological state of mind. Ironically, there are moments when we feel the need to be alone, as a matter of fact, some religious sects encourage their members to set themselves apart to enable them to reflect and meditate on their teachings.

Certain professionals also perform better when they are locked away from the public eye and away from all forms of distraction, yet, every year more and more people are said to suffer from loneliness.

Loneliness is a State of Mind

Loneliness is one of the human feelings that we all feel from time to time, for some, it is only a passing emotional feeling, for some others, it is a trigger for some undesirable and unpleasant feelings, the effect of which can be dire.

Loneliness can be described as a state of mine in which the individual feels alone or in a state of solitude. It causes the individual to feel empty, alone and undesired. Lonely individuals have a strong craving for human interaction, yet some of them have a personality that makes it difficult to form a connection with them. This deficiency in connecting has unfortunately not been solved even with more electronic gadgets and social media making communication easier, rather it seems to have aggravated it.

Psychologists have long found that as human beings, we have a strong desire for close relationships and social integration. It is because of reasons like this that loneliness is sometimes wrongly perceived as the absence of other humans around us, or lack of social integration yet there are many who live in the midst of people who feel totally alone. Many therapists have found that although a BPD may seem on the surface very outgoing, social, friendly with a capacity to strike conversations with anyone including strangers, they may still suffer from an acute case of loneliness.

There are many who spend a considerable amount of time feeling deeply alone in spite of the many acquaintances they have. The fact is, many of these lonely people have very few close friends and loved ones who really care about them, with that multitude of acquaintances only serving as social validations.

Being Alone Does Not Always Mean Being Lonely

Loneliness isn't necessarily about being alone, which can make it sometimes difficult to really diagnose because a person living alone and another who lives in the company of people can still feel lonely.

So, when next you see someone who parties hard, gets along easily with people, is charming, funny, and seems to have the best things in life on the outside, don't be in a hurry to beat yourself, they may just be trying to cover up or reduce the amount of time for them to be alone. You never know what goes in the closet and personal struggles of a lot of people away from prying eyes that is because they also have their own fair share of being stressed, anxious and depressed.

Beyond the surface level conversations, these people like the rest of us crave for deep levels of conversations, something many around them are unable to provide, which causes them to speak more freely with strangers who will not judge them and to create alternative profiles online where they can be free to express themselves.

Most celebrities are known victims of this.

Effects of Loneliness

Loneliness can affect your mental and physical health in a lot of ways, some of which are pretty obvious with others less obvious. The impact of loneliness when it affects major aspects of your body may not be known until they begin to manifest. What is however known is that, if you're lonely, you're more likely to be susceptible to various physical and mental ailments.

Loneliness Can Expose Your Heart to Risk

Loneliness raises your stress hormone levels so that your heart begins to work harder than it should, thereby increasing your blood pressure. Some of the unexplained high blood pressure and cardiovascular diseases can be traced to loneliness.

Loneliness Can Trigger Reduced Immunity

The immune system is the body's own mechanism of fighting off diseases and sickness that may want to affect the body. The stress hormones as a result of loneliness can cause the immune system of the body to malfunction and prevent it from performing its responsibility of fighting diseases and other illnesses.

Loneliness Can Trigger Inflammation in the Body

Many heart diseases stem from inflammation in the body, which can then result in cancer, Alzheimer, rheumatoid arthritis, and other heart diseases and loneliness is believed to be one of the triggers for them.

Sleeping Disorder

Sleep is one of the less obvious aspects of the human body that is affected by loneliness. People with sleep disorders wake up frequently at night, which reduces the quality of their sleep, resulting in the individual not resting enough.

The victims of such lose the physical and psychological restoration that they would have achieved from sleeping.

Loneliness Can Lead to Depression

Loneliness can lead to depression and depression can lead to loneliness, those two like to walk together like siblings. Not all loneliness will lead to depression, though, but being depressed is likely to be accompanied with loneliness.

Loneliness Increases the Risk of Suicide

Loneliness in itself is not likely to lead to suicidal tendencies, however, the effects of loneliness can make the victim lose self-esteem, feel unwanted, and depressed to the extent of wanting to end it all. Some also attempt suicide as a way of gaining attention from loved ones, who now have to pay extra care and attention to them.

Other indirect effects of loneliness can include:

- Alcoholism and drug abuse
- Reduction in memory and learning
- Increased Antisocial behavior
- Altered brain function
- Increased Cases of Poor decision-making

We all Are Lonely at Some Point in Life

As isolating as loneliness may seem, it is a normal human feeling that happens to everyone. We may feel lonely when a loved one is not available, separated, traveled, or deceased, which quickly passes away when the loved one or a replacement becomes available or time has healed the person. Social interaction in the form of friendship is a basic need of man, we depend on it for our mental health.

We are likely to feel lonely when we first move to a new city, change our neighborhood, break up with a friend or lover or exempted from a social gathering. We tend to be unhappy when faced with such isolation. In order for us to be happy, we need to share intimate bonds with our loved ones, people we can confide in, companions we can have a sense of belonging with, and a group of friends or family that we can give or get support from.

By now you should know that loneliness differs from being alone. While the former leaves us drained, upset and distracted, being alone as a result of desired solitude leaves us refreshed, at peace and creative.

Common Situations that can Make us Feel Alone

New Environment
You can feel lonely when you move into a new city where you do not know anyone or those you know are unavailable to keep you company. This can also happen if you are just starting out a new job, a new school or new church and have not made any acquaintances yet.

This feeling of being alone in this case is perfectly normal and is usually temporal. After a while, we get to know one person, then two and can eventually become a very popular person, but we probably started being alone.

The time between when we feel alone and when we begin to develop company differ from person to person. Some persons take much longer, while some hit the ground running as soon as they arrive at a new place.

Difference in Belief
This type of loneliness is usually associated with being in a situation when we are with people who do not share the same belief, culture, habits, and orientation as us. We may feel skeptical with joining them do what they do, it could be in the way they

worship that doesn't go down well with us so we can feel isolated.

We could also feel alone because of our sexual orientation. We may be afraid or ashamed to disclose our sexual orientation to our friends, family and loved ones which can further alienate us from these people which can make us feel lonely.

The absence of a Romantic Partner

There is the role of family and friends in our lives, there is also the role of a romantic partner either in the form of a lover, spouse or romantic partner. When such persons are unavailable or absent, perhaps for a short while, the tendency is for us to miss their presence, especially if we have gotten used to them.

The absence of a Loved Pet

Another situation that can lead to loneliness is when we are separated from a pet that we feel really attached to. This can happen when we go on a trip and are unable to take the pet along with us, it can also happen when the pet is dead.

It is not uncommon to have such feelings for our dogs, cats and other domestic pets. When these animals are not around, we can feel a sense of loss or something important being taken away from us.

Difference in Priorities

Sometimes, you may have friends who change their status and enter a new phase in their lives that change their priorities and vice versa. When that happens, we can find that they or you no longer have time for some of the things you all used to do. It could be because you or your friends got married, changed neighborhood, started a family, want to break a habit like smoking or got a new job.

We may also be in the midst of lots of acquaintances with quite lots of smiles, hellos, and pleasantries that do not go beyond the surface. With no one to have real conversations with, you are still going to feel alone despite being in the company of such people.

Another dimension to this could be when we are not quite sure of the sincerity of the friends we keep. If we do not feel that we can trust our friend's intentions to be true, helpful and with our interest in mind, we may begin to feel isolated from such people.

Loss of a Loved One

This is perhaps the most devastating known cause of loneliness. When we are separated from a person because of distance, we can always hope to be reunited with that person as soon as we can overcome that distance, but when it comes to death, the emotional feeling of such a loss can be catastrophic.

It could because of the death of a parent, friend, family member, roommate, lover or spouse. Some people never fully recover from such loss and carry the pain in their hearts for a long time. Some people, especially couples who are intimately attached to each other eventually pass on, not too long after the demise of their spouses.

Some kids have been known to mourn the loss of their parents many years after they have died, with many whose lives never remain the same. For a lot of others though, they are able to pull through the trying moments with a little help and support of friends, family, and other loved ones. Others are compelled to overcome their grief with the distraction of their daily life challenges. Luckily for such people, the healing effect of time is enough to see them through. There are those who, however only pull through with the help of therapists.

Whatever the case, loneliness will always exist in the world, whether we deliberately request for solitude or nature and circumstances imposes it on us.

Borderline Personality Disorder's Definition of Loneliness

While it is normal for many of us to avoid situations that make us feel lonely, those with borderline personality disorder have a disproportional fear of being alone that affects every aspect of their life. Borderline personality disorder (BPD) is considered one of the most serious mental illnesses that individuals can have especially with respect to how they interact with others around them and how they perceive being alone and abandoned. It tends to be characterized by pervasive mood instability and behaviors. Knowing what to look at for can help you know if you are dealing with someone with BPD.

If you have ever been with a person who exhibits qualities that fit into the following attributes, chances are that the person suffers from borderline personality disorder. Memoirs of their actions can help you keep track of your observations. This should however not serve as a replacement for proper diagnosis, as only a mental health care professional can diagnose a borderline personality disorder.

Symptoms of Borderline Personality Disorder

Although you are likely to observe varying symptoms of those with borderline personality disorder you come across, there are however some behaviors that are common to many of them. A few borderline personality disorder books have been able to document some of the symptoms that make understanding borderline personality disorder behavior a very interesting subject.

The most prominent of these behaviors is the extreme way they react to situations in which they correctly or incorrectly believe is going to leave them lonely as a result of being abandoned. Their reaction to minor disappointments, isolation, and rejection is usually extreme and intense. Because of their disproportionate fear of what can happen when they are not in the company of their friends, they act irrationally go into a cycle of breakups and makeups of their relationships and friendship with their loved one. They suffer from intense fear, anxiety, and shame even when there is no justifiable reason to do so.

Another feature to look out for in a borderline personality disorder is a history of instability in their relationships. They are very quick in changing from idealizing of their loved one, where they idolize this person with an intense expression of extreme love and then suddenly hating that lover intensely in what is known as devaluation. Their fear of loneliness also forces them to be overly dependent and reliant on friends, family members, spouse, and their lovers.

If you have personally encountered a BPD or read borderline personality disorder books, you will find that they are constantly scrutinizing their relationships for any sign of the other person abandoning them which increases their stress level with them ending most relationships almost as quickly as they start once there is any little problem, ironically, it is them who fear to be alone the most.

They can call you many times in a day just to try to ensure that you have not abandoned them even when they have nothing new to tell you in any of those calls.

The unfortunate outcome of this attitude is that they find themselves becoming lonely far quicker than they would have been if they did not harbor such fear. Their behavior drives away the very people who would have provided just the support they need so not to become lonely as they always fear.

For people with BPD, you will notice that there are no in-betweens, you are either totally good or totally bad. Everything is viewed from the viewpoint of extremity, as either idealization or devaluation, no room for anything between and these opinions do not take time in changing. They can suddenly become very angry or nervous and then excited or happy.

An individual who stayed late with them the previous day as a very passionate friend may be considered a traitor the very next morning, despite nothing happening to make them take up this new opinion. Then the very next day, they can call you up as if nothing happened and you are their best friend again. It is this inconsistency in their behavior that leads to instability in their relationships.

As humans, we tend to have idealized versions of ourselves, when we describe ourselves, we tend to talk about ourselves not really based on who we are, but based on who we wish to be. But for those with BPD, you will notice a pessimistic sign of the low self-value they place on themselves. They develop a distorted image of themselves that is frequently anxious about being loved and wanted, and then in their usual characteristics way of exhibiting extreme feelings, they perceive themselves of being worthless, unwanted and unloved.

This can be triggered by something as trivial as not first saying hello to them as soon as you entered a room in which they were other people present, or not calling them on the exact hour you promised not minding if you were busy at that time or were held back by a personal challenge.

One behavior many people who have had dealings with BPDs complain about is their tendency to indulge in impulsive and risky behavior that include indiscriminate sex, drug abuse, binge eating, driving recklessly and sometimes reckless shopping.

Their fear of loneliness can also lead them to blackmail their loved ones or friends not to leave them by indulging in self-harm and inflicting injuries on themselves. They also do not react well to criticism and strangely view disagreements and disappointments as an attempt to abandon them, a situation they find extremely difficult to handle.

Their behaviors are an indication of mood disorder and are considered dangerous enough to put them and others around them at risk. People with this problem suffer consistently from physical, psychological and emotional trauma resulting in conflicting and fluctuating impressions of who they are. One minute, they may view themselves as amazing individuals then the very next minute they may consider themselves as evil, unworthy and inadequate. They have issues with themselves and with everyone, finding it extremely difficult to cultivate and keep long-lasting relationships.

Their confusion leaves them empty, and unhappy, with no stable sense of who they are. They can trust a person wholeheartedly one minute and the next minute change their mind. Every second of the day is usually spent having the irrational fear of other people's intentions.

They are also in and out of suicidal thoughts, as frequently as the changes in their mood. In desperate situations, they are known to threaten suicide if they feel an individual they probably offended may be ditching them.

This display of unpredictable and erratic behavior can sometimes last for several days, at other times for just a few hours. Other behaviors exhibited by people with BPD include:

- Not able to empathize with others
- A tendency to be anxious and depressed
- Unable to keep steady jobs
- Display intense anger or problems controlling anger

The emotional disorder associated with BPD puts them in frequent painful mood swings that are beyond their control. What characterizes this disorder are the rapid and unpredictable changes that happen to their moods and behavior. They also suffer periods of hallucinations, stress, and depression. One of the most unfortunate ironies about BPD is that, although they intensely fear being abandoned, it is their behavior that causes others to eventual desert them.

Like other cases of mental health disorders, a person with BPD is likely to become exhausted with all the drama they exhibit. They are likely to feel drained by the constant up and downs associated with their mood swings, unstable behaviors, constant pessimism, and loneliness.

Causes of Borderline Personality Disorder

As with most mental health problems, Scientists are not exactly sure of what the causes of borderline personality disorder are, however, certain research seems to suggest that certain genes, environment, and social factors can trigger borderline personality disorder.

A History of Borderline Personality Disorder in the Family

Families that have had family members suffer from borderline personality disorder may have a higher risk of developing borderline personality disorder or at least exhibit a few traits of the disorder. This may be as a result of constant interaction with such individuals which can cause the person to begin to imitate or mirror some of the traits the victims' displays even though he himself may not like those behaviors. So, families that have borderline personality disorder parents, or borderline personality disorder in adolescents who are siblings, the probability tends to increase.

Changes in the Brain Structure
Persons with BPD are believed to have the problem as a result of certain structural and emotional changes in their brain sections that affect their control impulses and regulation of emotions. It is believed that this imbalance in the brain structure is what gives birth to this mental illness that becomes known as borderline personality disorder.

Environmental, Cultural, and Social Factors
Some other BPDs are made by situations they have faced in life which are traumatic in nature and inflicted on them by loved ones. The nature of these abuses can probably account for their lack of trust and also happen when they were abandoned, which also probably accounts for their fear of being abandoned.

They are usually victims of betrayed trust, child abuse, exposure to hostile conflicts, products of unstable relationships and victims of constant criticisms. Their troubled childhood tends to hunt them making them extremely insecure and constantly requiring validation.

While these factors are believed to increase the chances of a person developing BPD, there is no study to confirm that these factors will always trigger BPD. In short, there may be people without any of these factors who still go on to develop borderline personality disorder.

Effects Borderline Personality Disorder Instability on Loved Ones

The instability a borderline personality disorder friend or a borderline personality disorder lover can make a friendship or relationship with them an emotional battleground. This makes it difficult for anyone to have any meaningful relationship with them. BPD people tend to leave a long trail of emotional destruction along the way as they move on with life, having very few committed friends and many people who avoid them because of their attitude. A lot of patience and open-mindedness is also needed when dealing with people with BPD if you intend to have any meaningful and long term friendship with them.

Mental illnesses like this BPD creates a relationship that is likely to be consistently entrenched in conflict with the BPD individual always indulging in behaviors that puts a wedge between them and people around them. Friendships and relationships with BPD is usually a major point of impact and the effects of which do not delay in manifesting. Breaking up a normal relationship is hard in itself, but it is particularly more difficult when it comes to a victim with BPD.

The issues BPDs tend to react are usually a product of their negative creative imagination which constantly conjures up images of their loved one wanting to reject, abandon or betray them.

Talking to a Loved One with Borderline Personality

You will have to deal often with paranoia over very trivial issues some of them could be not picking up your phone on the first few rings. Their creative minds would probably conjure up an image of you being with another friend over them or you having an affair with your boss, hardly do they conjure up positive images of the possibility of you being in a meeting in that case.

One thing you will almost feel when dealing with them will be the amount of scrutiny you would be going through almost as if your friendship is being constantly tested with you having to always prove that you are a good friend or a faithful lover because of their tendency to always imagine the worst and waiting for you to confirm their worst fear at every time.

Many find that to be friends with them, you have to almost be a superman and of course, you will be rewarded with some moments of intense affection and love during the moments when they consider you the center of their world. The rules of engagement are usually going to be defined by them and also subject to change by them without notice.

Learning to Love Someone with Borderline Personality Disorder

It is tempting to imagine that they are just being delusional and a simple heart to heart talk will be sufficient to pull them out of the situation, unfortunately, that only works for a while with them going straight back to the same attitude not long after such chats. The emotions displayed by a BPD are genuine feelings that are very real to them. They are not feeling that you can talk them out of and cannot replace their perception with anything anyone tells them about their behavior.

Life with a BPD is a constant struggle, trying to understand their complex nature can leave you totally drained with your emotions running riot.

It is however not all gloom for people with BPD. There are men who are intrigued by women with BPD and are romantically drawn to the drama created by women who have this disorder. Perhaps the attention they get during periods of idealization compensates for those moments of devaluation. They also enjoy the dotting, attention, and drama that goes with BPD, which can make them feel special with the attention they get from and heroes when they rescue the BPD from their crisis.

Borderline Personality Disorder Parents

Parents of BPD also go through a lot when parenting BPD kids. They are usually the first victims of the tantrums in the behavior of their unstable BPD kids. Parents may also be forced to deal with the constant request for school change because of their perceived belief their teachers do not like them or their fellow students are not good enough. This can again be quickly followed by a change in the perception of the school, by describing it as one of the best schools in the locality with some of the best teachers and students.

A BPD can also show up at your workplace unannounced and disrupt a meeting you may be having with a colleague without considering the consequences to you or your career or even to them. To them at that time, their intense feeling overwhelms their sense of reasoning and all they want to do is to protect their territory so as not to be abandoned. Being involved with a BPD can cause your friends to also desert you. If you are very close to a BPD, it won't be long before you also begin to lose your friends the same way the BPD does.

Make Frequent Contacts with Them

If you are always willing to be available to a BPD, perhaps you could find ways to reduce the intense fear of abandonment they constantly feel of those close to them eventually deserting them. By providing them with the constant confirmation they desire to show that they really matter to you, you can help reduce the immense fear of abandonment they may have from your end.

The damage borderline personality disorder inflict on their loved ones can be devastating, fortunately, if they are willing they can seek the right kind of help. The least you can do for them is to point them in the direction of that help.

End it now if you are not cut out for drama

Now, this is not a textbook suggestion. Perhaps if you are not ready for this, you can skip this chapter and move to the next.

If you are not the kind of person who is cut out for unending drama with a highly dependent person who you may have to constantly reassure amidst all the inconsistency, then I have one advice for you, RUN, well, not run but you can also walk away. There are some people in life who, when we try to help them pull us down rather than us pulling them up, so before you decide to become the next savior of the world, it is in your best interest to seriously consider the consequences.

You Never Know What to Expect

Being friends or in a relationship with someone with borderline personality disorder will keep you shuttling between being loved and appreciated to being abandoned and hated. Even persons with BPD live a life that is constantly often filled with psychic pain which, when it becomes severe puts them at the borderline between reality and psychosis. So, if you happen to work in a school where you have to deal with borderline personality disorder in adolescent, you could also find yourself needing a borderline personality disorder survival guide because of the regular contact you are likely to have with them.

Lots of Psychological Stress Involved

The implication of these for those who associate with BPD people is that there will be a lot of distortion of perception. You will find yourself constantly staying in an environment that is toxic to you. Children who grow with borderline personality disorder parent tend to grow up with some level of low self-esteem after suffering from a lot of mental abuse from the parent who has the BPD. Husbands married to a BPD wife also find that loving a borderline personality disorder wife does not come easy.

If you do not want to be bombarded with unnecessary accusations, jealousy, and bullying, you are better off being away from them. If you decide to retain them as friends you may opt to minimize to as long as is reasonably possible for your interaction with them and the number of times you have to be around them. This is not you being mean, it is you taking precaution to ensure you do not descend into a mental case yourself. Their insecurity will cause them to try to control those around them, which will impress upon you great psychological stress to the extent of making you display some of their symptoms.

Lots of Drama mixed with the Storm

Yet many people will continue to delay the decision to move on with their lives. As dysfunctional and personally damaging friendship with BPD may be, some folks find it difficult to break through the cycle of repetition. We are all products of habits and find it difficult to get away from a situation we are familiar with, even if that situation is toxic to us. The feeling that you may have invested too much time to leave now may constantly play at the back of your mind.

Those who enjoy being in dramatic relationships, they could enjoy the ride in the storm in deriving excitements from the escapade of not knowing if the person who turns up is the idealizing one or the alter ego who devalues. They are a lot of things you are likely to experience being involved with BPDs, some of which will include:

• Leaving you completely drained with all their drama.

• Incapable of providing any emotional support in moments of your own needs

- The whole friendship will be all about them and on their own terms

- Their lack of progress as a result of their emotional instability

- You will always feel used and manipulated

- You'll always be on your toes daily, never knowing what to expect

- They can transfer their insecurity to you by constantly criticizing all your actions

One of the best things you can do for yourself will be to let them go. It will be one of the most important steps if you are interested in having a meaningful life yourself in future. That is because being constantly involved with them will prevent you from reaching your full potential. The complications and toxic drama they introduce at all times will weigh you down unnecessarily. Everyone who has succeeded in life will almost always speak of a support system that they relied on from time to time, a BPD will almost never fit into that role of a support system.

If you were to ever hesitate if you should leave BPD people or not, then perhaps knowing that they only help to bring out the worse in you may be able to convince you. Because of the bad habits, they tend to have in their moments of crisis, you would find yourself joining them in also having indiscriminate crazy sex, drinking and other unpalatable habits we discussed earlier. Just imagine your boss sees pictures of you being tagged in such pictures on social media.

Persons who have BPD will cause you to miss important aspects of your life. The emotional trauma you feel from the stress of being their friends will make you lose focus on important aspects of your life. Their instability and the negativity it brings will slowly, but surely begin to have its own impact on you. You could also begin to have panic attacks. You are going to miss appointments, meetings and interviews and even the ones you get to attend, you are probably going to be distracted most of the time because of the stress of being associated with a BPD.

Between being stretched thin by your sense of obligation, sympathy towards them, you will notice that your internal drive will begin to dwindle. The guilt and despair will impair your sense of judgment which will attract lots more miserable people to you.

So, for the sake of your own mental health, it will be in your best interest to begin to take steps to begin to leave. The case against keeping a BPD in your life is one you should not be taken likely, your life dreams, health could all become affected.

The experience of giving into their worries and the demands will very likely reduce your own brain activity, increase your risk of having heart diseases and an increase the chance of you dying early. The only way to protect yourself from the devastating physical, mental and emotional impact of being with BPD is to stay away from them as much as possible until they have gone to seek professional help and have begun to show significant improvement.

As social animals, we tend to attach a lot of importance to friendship. Our interaction with others has its own way of making us healthier, happier and increasing our self-esteem, contrary to what we will get from associating with BPDs.

By now you should be aware of the effects loving someone with borderline personality disorder can and will have on you, you can sense that you do not need them if you want to make any progress in life, the problem is you do not know how to leave them without the blackmail, drama and them hurting themselves. The first step will be for you to make the decision to let them go for your own good. If you are making the effort to leave and still can't take the bold step, then you should know that part of you yearns for the attention you get from them. You may also be under the influence of what is known as Stockholm syndrome. If you are not keeping them as an alibi for your own failure, something to blame in the future for your inability to make progress in life then now is the time to move on.

In spite of the need to leave a BPD, it is never an easy thing to do. Especially when we are in a relationship with them, it's not easy breaking up. Any unhealthy association, especially one that involves being associated with them comes with a lot of drama, you should expect more drama should you attempt to leave, because their most innate fears are predicated on you leaving and so they will pull all sorts of stunts, threaten to harm themselves and put the blame on you, if you leave them, but you will have to find a way to do it as quickly as possible and move on with your life.

Planning to Leave

Depending on how really involved you are with a BPD, you would have to do some level of thoughts and planning in your attempt to leave. You should ensure that the exit is done quickly without any drama from you. You also may want to consult a therapist that will help you deal with the emotional abuse you may have suffered been associated with a BPD. In some situations, the therapist may opt to help prepare the mind of the BPD to reduce the impact of your exit.

If the BPD is your spouse, such exits may require a greater level of planning. You probably would also be involving a lawyer in your case.

When you leave, you want it to be a permanent one, which means you should be taking all your possessions along with you. Your leaving should be total. You may have to ensure you remove any of your items at their place a little at a time so that they do not become suspicious, however, that is very hard to achieve because they are natural paranoia and do not require much evidence to trigger fear of being alone.

One other secret of BPD is that they tend to be on their best behaviors when in the presence of strangers. You can decide to use this to your advantage by announcing your intention to leave in the presence of strangers. If your association with them involves living under the same roof, then you may want to move out when they are not around.

You also do not want to be leaving a means of contacting you behind. You can out of courtesy call them from a public pay phone to let them know why they will not be seeing you anytime soon, but try not to leave a trace back to you. That may also mean alerting your mutual friends of your intention and possibly restricting their access to you so that they do not inadvertently lead the BPD back to you.

When You Finally Leave

When you leave and move on, make sure you really leave. You will have to ignore all the tantrums that will follow your exit. Most BPD are not necessarily bad people and there will be a lot of memories of the good times you had with them, but it will be in your best interest not to have any contact at all with them.

You will have to resist the anxiety and tension that may seem to overwhelm you. There will also be the possibility of experiencing post-traumatic stress disorder (PTSD) you probably would have grown accustomed to, which will as a habit continue to hunt you for a while until after a while when you may begin to notice the tension reducing and wearing away.

There will also probably be moments when you could possibly have feelings of doubts if you did the right thing or not by leaving them. You could probably be tempted to find out how they are doing, hoping that they are not doing anything extreme or hurting themselves. As mean as this may sound, now is not the time to look back. The BPD may also be trying to adjust, you should also let them go through their healing process in the best way they can without complicating the process for them.

Being associated with a BPD comes with a lot of drama, there will be that tendency to feel lonely without them around. You could possibly find that you are no longer used to having conventional friends having probably lost some of your old friends because of the BPD. You can, however, solve this by getting involved in other activities of interest, contact your old friend, making new friends, imbibing new hobbies, joining a club or even going back to school. You should, however, ensure you do not jump from one toxic situation to another.

An abandoned BPD partner can become dangerous and may want to retaliate by putting you in trouble with the authorities. They sometimes have the potential to harm themselves and point you out as suspects, which is why you should involve some level of support when breaking away from them.

Why it can be Hard to Leave a BPD Person

Being involved with a BPD and loving someone with a borderline personality disorder can have adverse effects on our mental health, yet for some people, rather than leave, they continuously stay in that relationship. Some of the reasons include:

The Periods of Idealization Excite Us

It can be hard to move away from a loving someone with a borderline personality disorder because of those good moments when they seem to be intensely into us and make us feel we are the next best thing to have happened to them. You could keep looking forward to such good moments of idealization that you do not realize the impact the fluctuation between idealization and devaluation can have on you.

False Sense of Improvement

You can also be attracted to those good moments which can make us believe that things can get better. You may see the good moments as moments of improvements which you may interpret as their willingness to change and get better.

Not wanting to hurt their feelings

You are likely to have a lot of soft spots for a BPD and probably also want to spare them the inevitable painful and uncomfortable conversation and how their reaction will be.

Fear of Loneliness

If the BPD is the only person you have around you, then you may also begin to feel afraid of being alone if you were to abandon the BPD. By constantly giving a lot of attention to the relationship as a way of avoiding conflict you could also be losing your independence. In that case, you desire to leave will not be as strong enough, as your perceived need to stay with what you are familiar with.

Staying to help

You may feel a sense of responsibility to them and want to help them get through the process, but the truth is, a BPD can only get better if they go through the right therapy, unfortunately, it is one of those things that can only succeed if they are willing to. The fact that they are some moments that seem good may trigger in you some hopes of being able to help them come with their situation.

TIPS FOR GETTING OUT IF YOU'RE STUCK with a BPD

You have to make a commitment

You have to make a decision once and for all that you're going to end it. Depending on how deeply involved you are with them, the process is not likely to be an easy one. You will probably need a lot of will power to see you through.

Make It Brief and Firm
There will be no need to drag things out. Attempting to break out in little steps will not only prolong the process, but it will also make it difficult for both you and the BPD to really make it happen.

Enlist the Support of Family and Friends
You should let your friends be aware of the situation in which you have found yourself and your desire to move on. Some members of your family can also be a sort of support base for you. However, the situation can be complicated if the person with the BPD is a member of your family like a parent or a sibling, then perhaps a different approach may be required. You should, however, create a safety net to help you get through this process. You should also be involving a therapist to guide you through the process.

Just Move on, Don't Try to be Friends
You should expect some form of drama and a lot of bad blood to happen after moving on with your life by abandoning the BPD. You should shove your friendship aside at this stage and focus on ensuring that you break free from the shackles of being their friend. That should be your primary focus for now.

Don't Try To Support the BPD Through the Process

As already stated, any contact with the BPD should be cut off. You do not want to be trying to rescue them during this period or trying to be their support system. You should also be aware of their attempt to blackmail and get you to come back again to them using various tricks that only them can conjure, you will have to call their bluff.

Engage in Meaningful Activities to Fill the void.

You will have to resist those moments when you feel the urge to call or contact a BPD you are trying to get rid of. To successfully do that especially in the early phase, you should spend your time in more positive ways and do things that make you feel good about yourself.

How to Patiently Care For Persons With Borderline Personality Disorder At Great Emotional Risk

While it is true that cutting off a BPD person is the most effective way to deal with them, the truth is, that solution is not always possible or practical. Sometimes, these people are not just ordinary friends, they could be our kids, parents or spouses. At that level of relationship, just walking away may not cut it for us, we may be compelled to care for them as well as try to help them.

They may also be friends who we feel obligated to help in one way or the other. We may also be in a relationship with a BPD that we are not willing to let go without as much as a fight, probably we assume that the issues are more of a relationship type rather than a mental health issue, whatever the reason, there are a few ways you can help.

However, before coming up with ways to help them, you should first learn how to live with them.

Living With A Borderline Personality Disorder

Be Predictable and Consistent

Borderline personality disorder is a serious mental disorder which results in vicious patterns of continuous mood instability, erratic behavior and a devalued image of one's self. These experiences often result in an inordinate fear of being abandoned which makes them act irrationally when they perceived any delay in action or inaction of yours to be a sign that you are leaving them.

To deal properly with that, you should endeavor to keep to your word, especially in matters relating to them. That means you should refuse to be swayed by their violent outburst, cries, blackmails with their tears, however, difficult it may be, for every time you give in to their outrage, the next episode becomes worse.

Encourage and Enforce Responsibility

Because of our closeness to the BPD, there will be the temptation to try to be the one who rescues them, what you should do is not to be manipulated into taking responsibilities for their irresponsible acts. Don't be the one who rushes out to bail them out all the time, they should learn to clean up their mess, whether it is when they assault someone at the mall, indulge in drunk driving, and any other irresponsible behavior. With no one to rescue them, they could begin to have an incentive to begin to change.

Keep All Arguments Short
Life with a BPD is always going to be filled with arguments, trying to correct a wrong impression because there will be many of them. Your genuine attempt to compliment and you could be accused of trying to patronize them. Every action has the potential to be misinterpreted and your actions perceived as not be concerned enough. When trying to clarify the situation you could find yourself involved in an endless argument, it is important to maintain a calm demeanor in such situations and allow it to ride out itself.

Family Guide to Borderline Personality Disorder

If you are a spouse or family member of someone with BPD, you may find yourself not knowing how to deal with the situation or reach to the emotional pain and abusive behavior of the BPD person with the situation looking hopeless and unbearable. The best possible way you can be of help to them is to seek mental health treatment for them from a qualified therapist. Couples and family members involved with BPD should be also involved in the treatment themselves so that the healing process can be quicker and have a more lasting effect. Experts believe that the BPD treatment is significantly enhanced if the treatment process includes the loved ones in it. The process will usually begin with all parties being educated on what the disorder is about and the type of skill set required to adequately deal with them and providing them with the support required for their emotional needs.

Being educated on BPD allows you to have a basic understanding of what to expect when involved with a BPD and how to quickly identify BPD behaviors. This education will help you learn how not to feel responsible for their actions as the BPD will try to make you feel for their emotional chaos and the crisis that follows.

You will find out that you will become better equipped to handle their manipulative behaviors and identify early signs of emotional outburst with a potential to leading to more serious problems as they begin to develop. Being aware will make it easier for both you and the BPD to learn to stop making these outbursts personal and identify them for what they truly are.

Many of those associated them with BPD tend to feel responsible for the emotional abuse they go through in the hands of a BPD. That is why a therapist will always try to provide some sort of validation and reassurance to the loved ones of a BPD about their own feelings which tends to be ignored by helping them remove the guilt they feel from them. You will learn that loving someone with borderline personality disorder is not easy.

As you struggle with understanding borderline personality disorder, you will learn that more than anything the BPD wants to be constantly reassured and validated. They earnestly want people to that are ready to constantly stay connected with them and making them feel wanted, loved and heard. Their emotional needs, however, tends to hinge almost always on blackmail.

The behavior of a BPD through their pattern of sabotaging friendship with their consistent pattern of over attachment and sudden abandonment will eventually exert a lot of stress on you which is why you should ensure you set very clear boundaries that they should not cross without consequences. Some of these boundaries may feel punitive, but for the benefit of the BPD and other occupants of the homes, maintaining a strict and consistent boundary will not only help the BPD, but it will also help reduce the mental torture others go through. This is usually not only about them, but also about the others who deserve to live a normal life.

The truth is, it is possible to live a healthy loving and normal life with a BPD, but it will take a lot of patience, persistence, love and supportive people. A lot of people have been able to successfully live healthy lives and live happily with BPD. It does come with a lot of sacrifices.

Conclusion

A person with a borderline personality disorder has an intense fear of what can happen to them in their loneliness which makes them very clingy and dependent on others for their self-health and validation. Their way of reacting to being lonely and abandoned is to drive the very people who can support them mad. Any slight disappointment sends a trigger to their mind that the person just like others is about to abandon and because they constantly have this fear in spite of the fact that there is no evidence to support it, they act in irrational manner that makes the other person really go away thereby confirming their initial fears which they carry on to the next victim.

Once you have identified a person as someone with a borderline personality disorder, you then need to make a decision if you want to stay on with them or continue showing them, love. A lot of people who are not interested in the drama associated with being with them simply cut off communicating with them and abandon them to pursue more serious things in life. Some follow them down the path for so long that leaving them becomes sort of difficult. These people sometimes find themselves sinking mentally and beginning to develop some of the symptoms of BPD and often also require therapy to stay sane.

There are those who as a result of being related to the BPD either as a borderline personality disorder parent, child, lover or spouse have to find a way to understand what the issues are and how best to live with them. These people sometimes out of love, sometimes out of obligation and other times feelings of responsibilities to them makes them want to stay and help them especially during their crisis.

With a lot of patience, sacrifice, love, and understanding, many people have been able to live with BPD patient and help them on their way to recovery.

One More Thing

If you enjoyed reading this book as much as I have enjoyed writing it, I'd appreciate if you can post a kind review on Amazon in the comments section.

Your comment can go a long way in convincing someone who is yet to decide.

Your support means a lot to me.

If you want to suggest ways of improvement, you can contact me here.

Thanks once again for taking your time to read this book.

Linsy